Excellence Despite

Mental Health

Struggles

By

Kristie Latasha Myers Short

Excellence Despite

Mental Health

Struggles

Kristie Latasha Myers Short

Copyright © 2018 by Kristie M. Short

Dedication

I give all the glory to God my Savior, to my lovely Mother Terry Myers, my husband, an all my Children thank you! Without your support and patience, I would not have achieved my goals.

Introduction

I am not a Doctor of education, but I can simply say despite mental health struggles you can strive for and be excellent in your endeavors. I struggled on various levels with mental situations and I received a diagnosis of bipolar in 1999.

Then and even today I am a loving, prudent wife, mother, daughter, Christian, and friend. I have been an LPN nurse for over 10 years.

My goal is not to write a novel of knowledge but to just help others. I enjoy Serving God, my husband, my children.

I'm not afraid to say I take medicines to stay balanced. A lot of people go wrong thinking medicines are weakness and they lack essential help. You don't have to let other thoughts control you to make you feel you can't succeed. Continue to dream! Don't let anyone kill your dreams regardless of your circumstances and illnesses.

Bipolar Face to Face

My name is Kristie Latasha Myers Short.
. I was born in Cheraw, S.C. I had an adventurous childhood. My Mom is fun-loving, caring, and hard-working and when I was about 3 yrs. Old Mom moved us to Bronx, NY. I was a happy and extremely funny; spoiled child. On special occasions I loved making silly faces with crazy noises. At the age of sixteen I gave my life to Christ. I became a more positive person by learning and obeying my bible.

When I was nineteen I met bipolar face to face or maybe mental health struggles is what I would say. Although I was in a battle, God would be right by my side. God of Noah, Abraham, and Isaac was holding my hand.

After my breakdown in 1998 at age 19,
 I stayed in the hospital for 3 weeks .
I thought my future was finished. After learning about mental health in psychology 101 , I never could imagine Having a mental illness. people would not understand, I didn't even understand myself or my situation.

After being diagnosed with bipolar. I thought what in the world is bipolar? Also, who are you to rename me that is not my name. After the attack I went back to work as a cashier. I became a candy stripper and I was taking courses at the technical College for Nursing. Some days I could not get out of the bed. My Mom was my inspiration, she would make me get out of the bed. People that knew me and my situation showered me with strange stares. In response I would just hold my head down and stare at the ground. I mean what could I.

I hate Medicines!

Then I had to take medicines. I hated medicines! The medicines made me slower and gain weight . As years went by bipolar tried to change me from a slim, confident, and joyful person to a large, insecure, and sad person. I could barely do simple things. I Mostly experienced mania than depression. I would talk a lot, make unwise choices, and have less patience. My symptoms are hard to notice because I am an extrovert. I would try to be perfect in my tasks. I would have a relapse mostly when my medicines were altered by the doctor.

The side effects would come. Some effects were weight gain, tiredness, blurred vision, dry mouth, excessive saliva, and other things. I continued to pray, to go to church, and read my bible. I asked God for a husband, nursing career, and children. My prayers were answered. I got married ,I have 3 children and I worked over 10 years as a nurse with bipolar.

Family Tree

I was told my Dad had a mental illness of some sort. I never would have been ashamed of my father. I once was ashamed of myself. I am more mature, and aware that I am not the only one.

My Mom oh how I love her. She was my super hero when I was drowning in insanity. She believes everything I say which at times was sometimes exaggerated. A mother's love can be dangerous if someone was messing with her babies. Picture a giant mother bear in that situation. Mom tried to help as much as she could. I was pushed away from her during those times.

I learned smart people do not neglect their mental health. They seek help as if it were their physical health. I have learned to love myself; craziness and all. I have struggled with taking my medicines. Sometimes I would feel groggy and drowsy.

I realized to stay healthy and out of the hospital that I needed my medicine. I learned this by experience. I learned by experience because I did not heed the doctor's advice. Living with this chemical imbalance I have learned so much. I learned how to live and love life. I have also learned to appreciate the small things.

Thank God for your mind each day. I have learned that I am not too good to take medication. Mental health disorders are not death sentences, they can be managed. You can still have happiness and a life. When medications take away the problem; to me that is a healing.

Mental Illness

My heart goes out to others with mental illnesses. Sometimes we cannot control some things about our lives. It's scary when a sickness controls your life.

God kept me in the past and today. He can do it for anyone. We need to trust him. Reading the bible helped me learn right thinking and serving Christ.

During Mania episodes I would argue with my adult loved ones and become distant, my words would be sharp and slicing. I thought everyone that was trying to help me were out to harm me .

I am normally full of love and smiles. I just praise the Lord for forgiveness, grace, and mercy that he has for us all . Illnesses try to bring out the ugly side of us. That is when we need to fight to be who we really are. Prayer was my greatest weapon.

Taking medicine was so tough. "I'm a Christian" " I'm a nurse" " I don't need" medicine I would say and think . Those sayings flooded my mind. I need medicine to help me be stable, a good Mom, and stable wife. Without my medication I could lose everything.

Remember "U"

Bipolar wanted to rename me. I'm still Kristie" tough. I feel beautiful still. Don't let bipolar, schizophrenia, depression, change you for the worst. I still strive today to do my best in all things .

Take care of your body and don't forget your mind, if you neglect these things you can't survive in this world You will not be here.

Galaxy of Madness

The disease tries to force you to be everything you are not. It is like an invisible fight to stay yourself. How can anyone participate in a fight when we can't see our opponent with our eyes. Jesus Christ fights for me. Otherwise. I probably would have been lost in the galaxy of madness.

I thankfully greet everyone with a smile each day. In others I see wonderings of lack of understanding how I can smile with an unpopular stigma. I learned I'm not subject only to my thoughts are others. It's Jesus thoughts that really matter. I have no reputation it is all about Jesus's reputation. I am also thankful that if someone don't understand bipolar, it's not my responsibility to make you.

I don't understand some things about it now. I did not ask for the disorder. I just try to live my life the best way possible. I also believe stress is a seed bipolar stem from.

After a setback or relapse, I never questioned my children's or husband's love for me.

I knew that they accepted me no matter what. We love to laugh, and so we laughed at me in the past crazy times, in this galaxy of madness. I talked to them a lot about it. The only time they were ashamed was when I would fuss at someone about my children. Otherwise I am an extremely fun and funny person. During setbacks I became very protective of my kids.

Managing Mental Disorder

My weight did increase. I craved carbs. I have learned with adequate exercise and healthy choices you can lose weight. At first, I was so worried about my reputation. I went to mental hospitals several times. Now I have learned to much stress can produce abnormal behaviors in anyone. I saw some of my coworkers at the hospitals. The hospitals help your physical and mental health. It is sad some people refuse help that they really need. I enjoyed meeting and encouraging others. The food was awesome.

You must take control of your thoughts to be stable with bipolar. You may even change your mind and moods a lot. Learn stability in every stage of your life. Practice thinking positive thoughts.

Pray for God's help because that can be tough. Study the bible . As a parent of 3 children I pray often throughout the day. Sometimes little things such as the kids messing up could irritate me. So, I practice being slow to anger and quick to show love and patience. I take quiet breaks also I exercise to release stress. Keeping the House Organized can keep your thoughts organized.

You can still be happy with bipolar. Yes, you can . It is a manageable disorder. Someone could have had your bipolar life and you not exist. Or you could have had something worse than bipolar.

Always :

- Keep your goals and dreams.
- Put God first
- Then take one day at a time.
- Love and be kind to your family.
- Stay thankful for their support.
- Some people can work with bipolar.
- Take one day at time.

Hospital Visits

I had to go to the hospital on occasions Most of the time I was not self-volunteered but committed. I can finally talk about it because it can help someone else. Maybe that's why I went through it to start off with.

I met and saw many interesting people. Some had eating disorders, major depression, bipolar, schizophrenia, and much more. Everyone had a story to tell. The food was so good. We always looked forward to meals at one hospital you made your means and ate as much as possible. I had lost weight coming in and gained it back going out.

My favorite hospital was McLeod hospital in Florence, South Carolina. They had the best food, exercising machines, the most phone time, good groups, an atmosphere. They also had caring nurses. Some situations were so funny I said to a nurse "what am I doing here?

And cried laughing. I mean one lady said on the phone to her husband "I don't have no pants no socks, no shirts, no underclothing, what you do all day, I have no clothes packed inside the suitcase. I love to laugh, and I do so easily. I ran away to my room to laugh. I saw God change and heal some of the people there. It's amazing the positive effects of the medicine. One guy was enjoying the food so well he didn't know that he was in the mental hospital after 5 days.

Also, side effects of the medicine can be troublesome. I deal with mild neck twitching and arm stiffness occasionally, but I'm sane. I can still do what I need such as drive, take care of my family, without meds I'm a disarray of confusion and chaos. I accept this part of my being now and I love "Kristie" I'm still beautiful inside and out.

Although I can act ugly at times without the medicine, God allowed me to go through this. We all act ugly at times. That is the humanity in us all. I'm in much need of the fruit of the sprit self-control. I know God can do all and above what we think or even ask.

The joke is really on you when laugh at others taking medicines for mental health. The medicines help them do what they need to do. Can you tolerate medicine working against your will and still get your duties done?

I never knew I would battle with bipolar. Everybody can't beat bipolar, can you? It is like someone or something you can't see that tries to steal your prized possessions such as your personality, talents, and traits. It tries to steal the things that make you yourself. How would you fight bipolar? Jesus Christ teaches me how to fight this invisible enemy.

Dealing with mental health I was so hungry for encouragement, guidance, and knowledge. I want to be available to others with my experience. Most of the time I received mean also judgmental stares, as if I asked for the illness. Others watched me as a hawk waiting for a relapse. I could see rejoicing in some of their eyes as I was drowning in despair. There were ones who were calm, quiet, and kind. When I heard stories of real peoples' experiences, it was like stepping stones in my life to go on.

I encouraged myself that this is my only life on earth, so I was not going to let mental illness steal my working ability, my time, or my life. It tried to take over thing it could. My reason for this book is to help those who are down . Some people kick people when they are down. I know how it feels to need a hug, smile, encouragement or prayer. This world is full of criticism and judging. Love is rare, ancient; but powerful and much needed. It can even cause change. It is a blessing to have a heart that can love.

This sickness taught me how to live better and enjoy my blessings. Most people with mental health problems are very talented. I truly believe we use more than 10% of our brains. Sadly, to say I believe some of us have been chemically abused with meds. Sometimes I feel a guinea pig or science rat. I met all types of people in the hospitals some with mild and extreme disorders and diagnosis. One thing I learned all conditions or illnesses were as different as personalities, so Doctors can not treat them the same.

Poetry

by KLMS

It's Time to Shine

I have been in the dark so long, I'm ready to glow

The writer's block is gone now and it's time to flow

I have to release the pain and let my emotions go

My body is not old anymore even my mind is new

I'm going to talk can't keep it in

That was the past now let the future begin!

Depression

By KLMS

It comes down and rest over you like a cloud

It can be heavy or mild

It befriends you after a sickness, failure, or death

It may try to come back even after it has left

God's power is the light to this dark spirit

He has all the victory no reason to fear it.

My Healing

By KLMS

It seemed as if I was down so long

I couldn't get up the sickness was to
strong

Bipolar tried to steal who I was and
wanted to be

I couldn't even take care of my family

No I did not have the strength to do it on
my own

God was my strength I was not alone

Bipolar threaten to steal my talents, joy,
and peace

But God said "Release"!

I thought I could not be healed by
medicine

But I'm on medicine and the healing has
just begun

About the Author

Krishe Myers Short is the mother of three children, Shemaiah Ulani Short, Stephon Khalil Short, and Sierra Aliyah Short. She has been married to Tony Short for 18yrs. She is a LPN Nurse. She has been nursing for 15 yrs.

The purpose of this book is to give God the glory, with God all things are possible. Al so to encourage others. she has started a support group . Kristie resides in South Carolina

Kshort30@yahoo.com